baby's first months
with Sophie la girafe®

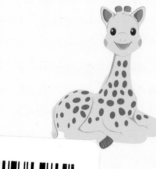

D0009563

THE EXPERIMENT

BECAUSE EVERY BOOK IS A TEST OF NEW IDEAS

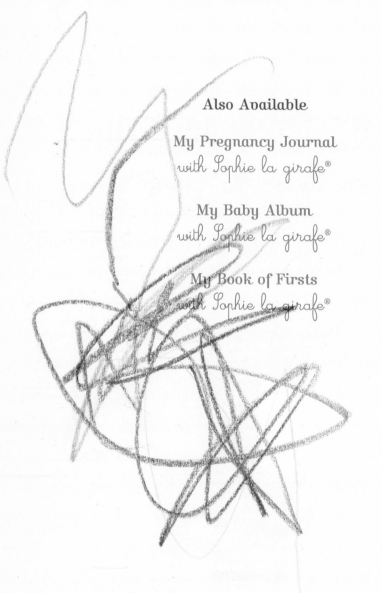

baby's first months
with Sophie la girafe®

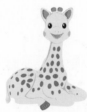

a daily log book

THE EXPERIMENT
NEW YORK

Enjoy the ride

Your baby is here!

Your newborn's arrival brings not only incredible upheaval but also incredible joy. You'll want to remember everything—baby's first laugh, first smile, and the first time her little fingers latched on to yours. But before you can remember the precious times, you have to make it through the first few weeks of change.

You constantly wake up to baby's nightly fussing (or bawling!), the day is a long line of feedings, you have to carefully plan outings around nap time, and you feel like a diaper-changing machine.

So how do you deal with those first few weeks and months when you're so tired you can barely put a sentence together and when day and night blur into one? This journal will help you take a step back and get organized. As the days go by, it will help you keep track, all in one place. You can record everything about your baby's daily life with specific information about baby's schedule such as meals, changings, sleep times, and crying. Note down anything and everything—including how you're feeling! You'll quickly see the benefits:

- You can give your doctor reliable information
- You can share information with other caregivers
- You'll understand your baby's needs much faster
- Over time, you'll see your baby progress to a more consistent schedule: how reassuring!

The life of a parent is anything but boring! As long as you keep smiling, you and your baby can enjoy the ride.

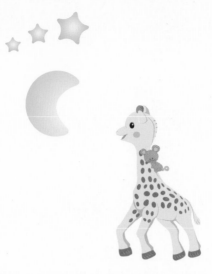

Good night and sleep tight!

All new parents obsess over when their baby will sleep through the night. Take heart: At some point in the first year, your baby will start sleeping for about 10 hours each night.

Every child is different, though. When your baby first arrives home, he may sleep for 16 or more hours a day, often in stretches of just a few hours at a time. As he matures and can go longer between feedings, you'll find a more consistent sleep pattern.

Day/night

For newborns, "sleeping through the night" means getting used to their internal body clocks. The goal is to help your baby tell the difference between day and night and give her clear signals between these two periods.

This means . . .

Daytime

- Keep your baby awake by talking to him or singing songs

- Chat with your baby during meals and wake him up if he falls asleep while eating

- Avoid keeping the house too dark or quiet during nap time

Nighttime

- Avoid keeping the light too bright during a feeding

- Let your baby fall asleep, even during a feeding

- Speak softly especially during changings

Keep a routine!

A routine will help your baby eat at regular hours and sleep through the night, every night, and this journal will help you create one. Repeated actions and small habits like a soft lullaby, reading from a picture book, and a kiss on the eyes will create a good sleeping environment and signal to your baby that it's time for bed.

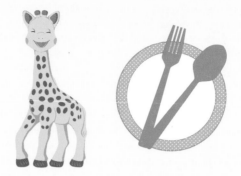

Eating enough to grow!

Is your baby getting enough milk? Will she grow big and strong? Regular visits to the doctor will answer your questions and reassure you. Keep track of weight, length, and immunizations with the charts in this book. Weight milestones in the first few weeks will indicate if your baby should be woken up to feed. But how will you know on a daily basis if baby is eating enough?

Your baby's schedule will evolve over time, and this is perfectly normal. At first, your baby will need 8 to 12 feedings a day (about one feeding every 2 to 3 hours). Important signs that your newborn is getting enough food include: steady weight gain, contentment between feedings, and wetting at least 6 diapers a day.

Bottle feeding

Use this journal to note down when your baby feeds, and, if you're bottle feeding (whether with breast milk or formula), how much he drinks so that you can track his daily intake. Newborns consume about 1.5 to 3 ounces at each feeding; at two months babies may consume 4 to 5 ounces at each feeding. You and your doctor can decide whether he's getting too much or too little.

Breastfeeding

When you breastfeed, you can never tell exactly how much milk your baby is getting, but you can keep track of how long baby feeds. As time goes on, breast milk production will increase; depending on the volume of milk created your baby may need to feed less often or more often. Note the start time and end time of each feeding or set a timer to track the duration. Note which breast you use each time to avoid engorgement and infection—drain the first breast and switch to the next if baby is still hungry or start the next feeding with the other breast. Breast pumping helps increase milk production, will give you an idea of the volume of milk you're producing, and keeps baby fed while you're away.

Dirty diapers

In addition to weight gain, you can tell whether your baby is getting enough to eat from her diaper changes, which is why you need to keep track of them. Your baby is feeding enough if she wets 6 to 8 diapers every 24 hours. Note if the color, consistency, and frequency of poopy diapers changes—not pleasant, but these are important details to be aware of, and to relay to your doctor.

Listen to your baby

Your crying baby is just trying to tell you something—the more attuned you are to his schedule and needs, the easier it is to decipher his cries. Stirring, stretching, sucking motions, and lip movements can be early indicators of hunger—by watching for them, you can help to avoid your baby starting to wail! By keeping clear track of feedings, sleep, diaper changes, fussing, and crying you can pick up on patterns to help you better respond to your baby's needs.

Important contacts

Personal contacts

_____ (parent)

....

....

_____ (parent)

....

....

Other contacts (grandparents, babysitter, other family, friends)

....

....

....

....

....

Doctor

....

....

....

....

....

Emergency numbers

Pediatric emergency:

....

Local emergency room:

....

Police department:

....

Fire department:

....

Growth

Date	Weight (pounds & ounces)	Length (inches)	Head (inches)	Percentile (percent)

Immunizations

Vaccines	Disease	Date	Date	Date	Date
HepB	hepatitis B				
RV	rotavirus				
DTaP	Tetanus, pertussis (whooping cough), and diphtheria				
Hib	haemophilus influenza type b				
PCV	pneumococcus				
IPV	polio				
Flu	influenza				
MMR	measles, mumps, and rubella				
Varicella	chickenpox				
HepA	hepatitis A				

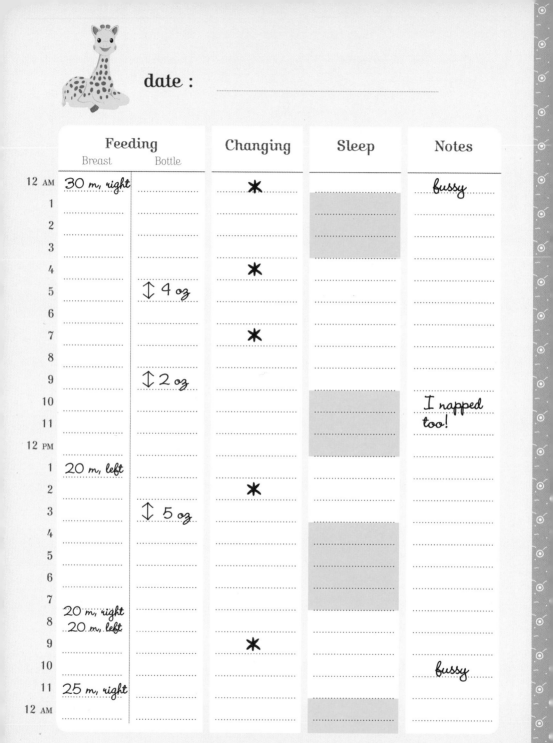

date : ....

	Feeding		Changing	Sleep	Notes
	Breast	Bottle			
12 AM	30 m, right		✳		fussy
1					
2					
3					
4			✳		
5		↕ 4 oz			
6					
7			✳		
8					
9		↕ 2 oz			
10					I napped
11					too!
12 PM					
1	20 m, left				
2			✳		
3		↕ 5 oz			
4					
5					
6					
7	20 m, right				
8	20 m, left				
9			✳		
10					fussy
11	25 m, right				
12 AM					

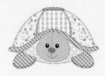

date : ....

	Feeding		Changing	Sleep	Notes
	Breast	Bottle			
12 AM	....	....	....	....	....
1	....	....	....	....	....
2	....	....	....	....	....
3	....	....	....	....	....
4	....	....	....	....	....
5	....	....	....	....	....
6	....	....	....	....	....
7	....	....	....	....	....
8	....	....	....	....	....
9	....	....	....	....	....
10	....	....	....	....	....
11	....	....	....	....	....
12 PM	....	....	....	....	....
1	....	....	....	....	....
2	....	....	....	....	....
3	....	....	....	....	....
4	....	....	....	....	....
5	....	....	....	....	....
6	....	....	....	....	....
7	....	....	....	....	....
8	....	....	....	....	....
9	....	....	....	....	....
10	....	....	....	....	....
11	....	....	....	....	....
12 AM	....	....	....	....	....

date : ....

	Feeding		Changing	Sleep	Notes
	Breast	Bottle			
12 AM	....	....	....	....	....
1	....	....	....	....	....
2	....	....	....	....	....
3	....	....	....	....	....
4	....	....	....	....	....
5	....	....	....	....	....
6	....	....	....	....	....
7	....	....	....	....	....
8	....	....	....	....	....
9	....	....	....	....	....
10	....	....	....	....	....
11	....	....	....	....	....
12 PM	....	....	....	....	....
1	....	....	....	....	....
2	....	....	....	....	....
3	....	....	....	....	....
4	....	....	....	....	....
5	....	....	....	....	....
6	....	....	....	....	....
7	....	....	....	....	....
8	....	....	....	....	....
9	....	....	....	....	....
10	....	....	....	....	....
11	....	....	....	....	....
12 AM	....	....	....	....	....

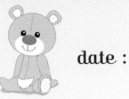

date : ....

	Feeding		Changing	Sleep	Notes
	Breast	Bottle			
12 AM					
1					
2					
3					
4					
5					
6					
7					
8					
9					
10					
11					
12 PM					
1					
2					
3					
4					
5					
6					
7					
8					
9					
10					
11					
12 AM					

date : ....

	Feeding		Changing	Sleep	Notes
	Breast	Bottle			
12 AM	....	....	....	....	....
1	....	....	....	....	....
2	....	....	....	....	....
3	....	....	....	....	....
4	....	....	....	....	....
5	....	....	....	....	....
6	....	....	....	....	....
7	....	....	....	....	....
8	....	....	....	....	....
9	....	....	....	....	....
10	....	....	....	....	....
11	....	....	....	....	....
12 PM	....	....	....	....	....
1	....	....	....	....	....
2	....	....	....	....	....
3	....	....	....	....	....
4	....	....	....	....	....
5	....	....	....	....	....
6	....	....	....	....	....
7	....	....	....	....	....
8	....	....	....	....	....
9	....	....	....	....	....
10	....	....	....	....	....
11	....	....	....	....	....
12 AM	....	....	....	....	....

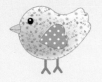

date :

	Feeding		Changing	Sleep	Notes
	Breast	Bottle			
12 AM					
1					
2					
3					
4					
5					
6					
7					
8					
9					
10					
11					
12 PM					
1					
2					
3					
4					
5					
6					
7					
8					
9					
10					
11					
12 AM					

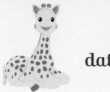

date : ....

	Feeding		Changing	Sleep	Notes
	Breast	Bottle			
12 AM					
1					
2					
3					
4					
5					
6					
7					
8					
9					
10					
11					
12 PM					
1					
2					
3					
4					
5					
6					
7					
8					
9					
10					
11					
12 AM					

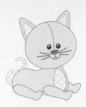

date :

	Feeding		Changing	Sleep	Notes
	Breast	Bottle			
12 AM					
1					
2					
3					
4					
5					
6					
7					
8					
9					
10					
11					
12 PM					
1					
2					
3					
4					
5					
6					
7					
8					
9					
10					
11					
12 AM					

date : ....

	Feeding		Changing	Sleep	Notes
	Breast	Bottle			
12 AM					
1					
2					
3					
4					
5					
6					
7					
8					
9					
10					
11					
12 PM					
1					
2					
3					
4					
5					
6					
7					
8					
9					
10					
11					
12 AM					

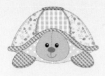

date : ....

	Feeding		Changing	Sleep	Notes
	Breast	Bottle			
12 AM					
1					
2					
3					
4					
5					
6					
7					
8					
9					
10					
11					
12 PM					
1					
2					
3					
4					
5					
6					
7					
8					
9					
10					
11					
12 AM					

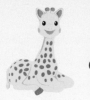

date : ....

	Feeding		Changing	Sleep	Notes
	Breast	Bottle			
12 AM					
1					
2					
3					
4					
5					
6					
7					
8					
9					
10					
11					
12 PM					
1					
2					
3					
4					
5					
6					
7					
8					
9					
10					
11					
12 AM					

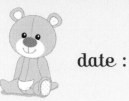

date : ....

	Feeding		Changing	Sleep	Notes
	Breast	Bottle			
12 AM					
1					
2					
3					
4					
5					
6					
7					
8					
9					
10					
11					
12 PM					
1					
2					
3					
4					
5					
6					
7					
8					
9					
10					
11					
12 AM					

date : ....

	Feeding		Changing	Sleep	Notes
	Breast	Bottle			
12 AM					
1					
2					
3					
4					
5					
6					
7					
8					
9					
10					
11					
12 PM					
1					
2					
3					
4					
5					
6					
7					
8					
9					
10					
11					
12 AM					

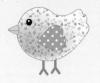

date : ....

	Feeding		Changing	Sleep	Notes
	Breast	Bottle			
12 AM					
1					
2					
3					
4					
5					
6					
7					
8					
9					
10					
11					
12 PM					
1					
2					
3					
4					
5					
6					
7					
8					
9					
10					
11					
12 AM					

date : ....

	Feeding		Changing	Sleep	Notes
	Breast	Bottle			
12 AM					
1					
2					
3					
4					
5					
6					
7					
8					
9					
10					
11					
12 PM					
1					
2					
3					
4					
5					
6					
7					
8					
9					
10					
11					
12 AM					

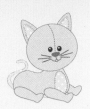

date :

	Feeding		Changing	Sleep	Notes
	Breast	Bottle			
12 AM					
1					
2					
3					
4					
5					
6					
7					
8					
9					
10					
11					
12 PM					
1					
2					
3					
4					
5					
6					
7					
8					
9					
10					
11					
12 AM					

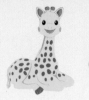

date :

	Feeding		Changing	Sleep	Notes
	Breast	Bottle			
12 AM					
1					
2					
3					
4					
5					
6					
7					
8					
9					
10					
11					
12 PM					
1					
2					
3					
4					
5					
6					
7					
8					
9					
10					
11					
12 AM					

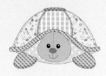

date : ....

	Feeding		Changing	Sleep	Notes
	Breast	Bottle			
12 AM					
1					
2					
3					
4					
5					
6					
7					
8					
9					
10					
11					
12 PM					
1					
2					
3					
4					
5					
6					
7					
8					
9					
10					
11					
12 AM					

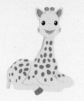

date :

	Feeding		Changing	Sleep	Notes
	Breast	Bottle			
12 AM					
1					
2					
3					
4					
5					
6					
7					
8					
9					
10					
11					
12 PM					
1					
2					
3					
4					
5					
6					
7					
8					
9					
10					
11					
12 AM					

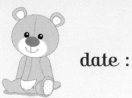

date : ....

	Feeding		Changing	Sleep	Notes
	Breast	Bottle			
12 AM					
1					
2					
3					
4					
5					
6					
7					
8					
9					
10					
11					
12 PM					
1					
2					
3					
4					
5					
6					
7					
8					
9					
10					
11					
12 AM					

date : ....

	Feeding		Changing	Sleep	Notes
	Breast	Bottle			
12 AM					
1					
2					
3					
4					
5					
6					
7					
8					
9					
10					
11					
12 PM					
1					
2					
3					
4					
5					
6					
7					
8					
9					
10					
11					
12 AM					

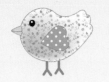

date : ....

	Feeding		Changing	Sleep	Notes
	Breast	Bottle			
12 AM					
1					
2					
3					
4					
5					
6					
7					
8					
9					
10					
11					
12 PM					
1					
2					
3					
4					
5					
6					
7					
8					
9					
10					
11					
12 AM					

date : ....

	Feeding		Changing	Sleep	Notes
	Breast	Bottle			
12 AM					
1					
2					
3					
4					
5					
6					
7					
8					
9					
10					
11					
12 PM					
1					
2					
3					
4					
5					
6					
7					
8					
9					
10					
11					
12 AM					

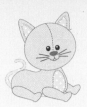

date : ....

	Feeding		Changing	Sleep	Notes
	Breast	Bottle			
12 AM					
1					
2					
3					
4					
5					
6					
7					
8					
9					
10					
11					
12 PM					
1					
2					
3					
4					
5					
6					
7					
8					
9					
10					
11					
12 AM					

date : ....

	Feeding		Changing	Sleep	Notes
	Breast	Bottle			
12 AM					
1					
2					
3					
4					
5					
6					
7					
8					
9					
10					
11					
12 PM					
1					
2					
3					
4					
5					
6					
7					
8					
9					
10					
11					
12 AM					

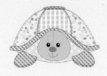

date : ....

	Feeding		Changing	Sleep	Notes
	Breast	Bottle			
12 AM					
1					
2					
3					
4					
5					
6					
7					
8					
9					
10					
11					
12 PM					
1					
2					
3					
4					
5					
6					
7					
8					
9					
10					
11					
12 AM					

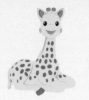

date : ....

	Feeding		Changing	Sleep	Notes
	Breast	Bottle			
12 AM					
1					
2					
3					
4					
5					
6					
7					
8					
9					
10					
11					
12 PM					
1					
2					
3					
4					
5					
6					
7					
8					
9					
10					
11					
12 AM					

date :

	Feeding		Changing	Sleep	Notes
	Breast	Bottle			
12 AM					
1					
2					
3					
4					
5					
6					
7					
8					
9					
10					
11					
12 PM					
1					
2					
3					
4					
5					
6					
7					
8					
9					
10					
11					
12 AM					

date : ....

	Feeding		Changing	Sleep	Notes
	Breast	Bottle			
12 AM					
1					
2					
3					
4					
5					
6					
7					
8					
9					
10					
11					
12 PM					
1					
2					
3					
4					
5					
6					
7					
8					
9					
10					
11					
12 AM					

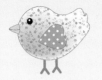

date : ....

	Feeding		Changing	Sleep	Notes
	Breast	Bottle			
12 AM					
1					
2					
3					
4					
5					
6					
7					
8					
9					
10					
11					
12 PM					
1					
2					
3					
4					
5					
6					
7					
8					
9					
10					
11					
12 AM					

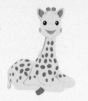

date : ....

	Feeding		Changing	Sleep	Notes
	Breast	Bottle			
12 AM					
1					
2					
3					
4					
5					
6					
7					
8					
9					
10					
11					
12 PM					
1					
2					
3					
4					
5					
6					
7					
8					
9					
10					
11					
12 AM					

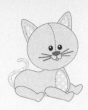

date : ....

	Feeding		Changing	Sleep	Notes
	Breast	Bottle			
12 AM					
1					
2					
3					
4					
5					
6					
7					
8					
9					
10					
11					
12 PM					
1					
2					
3					
4					
5					
6					
7					
8					
9					
10					
11					
12 AM					

date :

	Feeding		Changing	Sleep	Notes
	Breast	Bottle			
12 AM					
1					
2					
3					
4					
5					
6					
7					
8					
9					
10					
11					
12 PM					
1					
2					
3					
4					
5					
6					
7					
8					
9					
10					
11					
12 AM					

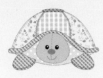

date : ....

	Feeding		Changing	Sleep	Notes
	Breast	Bottle			
12 AM	....	....	....	....	....
1	....	....	....	....	....
2	....	....	....	....	....
3	....	....	....	....	....
4	....	....	....	....	....
5	....	....	....	....	....
6	....	....	....	....	....
7	....	....	....	....	....
8	....	....	....	....	....
9	....	....	....	....	....
10	....	....	....	....	....
11	....	....	....	....	....
12 PM	....	....	....	....	....
1	....	....	....	....	....
2	....	....	....	....	....
3	....	....	....	....	....
4	....	....	....	....	....
5	....	....	....	....	....
6	....	....	....	....	....
7	....	....	....	....	....
8	....	....	....	....	....
9	....	....	....	....	....
10	....	....	....	....	....
11	....	....	....	....	....
12 AM	....	....	....	....	....

date : ....

	Feeding		Changing	Sleep	Notes
	Breast	Bottle			
12 AM	....	....	....	....	....
1	....	....	....	....	....
2	....	....	....	....	....
3	....	....	....	....	....
4	....	....	....	....	....
5	....	....	....	....	....
6	....	....	....	....	....
7	....	....	....	....	....
8	....	....	....	....	....
9	....	....	....	....	....
10	....	....	....	....	....
11	....	....	....	....	....
12 PM	....	....	....	....	....
1	....	....	....	....	....
2	....	....	....	....	....
3	....	....	....	....	....
4	....	....	....	....	....
5	....	....	....	....	....
6	....	....	....	....	....
7	....	....	....	....	....
8	....	....	....	....	....
9	....	....	....	....	....
10	....	....	....	....	....
11	....	....	....	....	....
12 AM	....	....	....	....	....

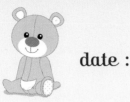

date : ....

	Feeding		Changing	Sleep	Notes
	Breast	Bottle			
12 AM					
1					
2					
3					
4					
5					
6					
7					
8					
9					
10					
11					
12 PM					
1					
2					
3					
4					
5					
6					
7					
8					
9					
10					
11					
12 AM					

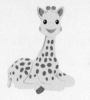

date : ....

	Feeding		Changing	Sleep	Notes
	Breast	Bottle			
12 AM					
1					
2					
3					
4					
5					
6					
7					
8					
9					
10					
11					
12 PM					
1					
2					
3					
4					
5					
6					
7					
8					
9					
10					
11					
12 AM					

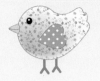

date : ....

	Feeding		Changing	Sleep	Notes
	Breast	Bottle			
12 AM					
1					
2					
3					
4					
5					
6					
7					
8					
9					
10					
11					
12 PM					
1					
2					
3					
4					
5					
6					
7					
8					
9					
10					
11					
12 AM					

date : ....

	Feeding		Changing	Sleep	Notes
	Breast	Bottle			
12 AM					
1					
2					
3					
4					
5					
6					
7					
8					
9					
10					
11					
12 PM					
1					
2					
3					
4					
5					
6					
7					
8					
9					
10					
11					
12 AM					

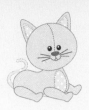

date : ....

	Feeding		Changing	Sleep	Notes
	Breast	Bottle			
12 AM					
1					
2					
3					
4					
5					
6					
7					
8					
9					
10					
11					
12 PM					
1					
2					
3					
4					
5					
6					
7					
8					
9					
10					
11					
12 AM					

date : ....

	Feeding		Changing	Sleep	Notes
	Breast	Bottle			
12 AM					
1					
2					
3					
4					
5					
6					
7					
8					
9					
10					
11					
12 PM					
1					
2					
3					
4					
5					
6					
7					
8					
9					
10					
11					
12 AM					

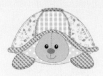

date : ....

	Feeding		Changing	Sleep	Notes
	Breast	Bottle			
12 AM	....	....	....	....	....
1	....	....	....	....	....
2	....	....	....	....	....
3	....	....	....	....	....
4	....	....	....	....	....
5	....	....	....	....	....
6	....	....	....	....	....
7	....	....	....	....	....
8	....	....	....	....	....
9	....	....	....	....	....
10	....	....	....	....	....
11	....	....	....	....	....
12 PM	....	....	....	....	....
1	....	....	....	....	....
2	....	....	....	....	....
3	....	....	....	....	....
4	....	....	....	....	....
5	....	....	....	....	....
6	....	....	....	....	....
7	....	....	....	....	....
8	....	....	....	....	....
9	....	....	....	....	....
10	....	....	....	....	....
11	....	....	....	....	....
12 AM	....	....	....	....	....

date : ....

	Feeding		Changing	Sleep	Notes
	Breast	Bottle			
12 AM					
1					
2					
3					
4					
5					
6					
7					
8					
9					
10					
11					
12 PM					
1					
2					
3					
4					
5					
6					
7					
8					
9					
10					
11					
12 AM					

date : ....

	Feeding		Changing	Sleep	Notes
	Breast	Bottle			
12 AM					
1					
2					
3					
4					
5					
6					
7					
8					
9					
10					
11					
12 PM					
1					
2					
3					
4					
5					
6					
7					
8					
9					
10					
11					
12 AM					

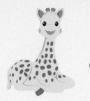

date :

	Feeding		Changing	Sleep	Notes
	Breast	Bottle			
12 AM					
1					
2					
3					
4					
5					
6					
7					
8					
9					
10					
11					
12 PM					
1					
2					
3					
4					
5					
6					
7					
8					
9					
10					
11					
12 AM					

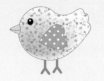

date : ....

	Feeding		Changing	Sleep	Notes
	Breast	Bottle			
12 AM					
1					
2					
3					
4					
5					
6					
7					
8					
9					
10					
11					
12 PM					
1					
2					
3					
4					
5					
6					
7					
8					
9					
10					
11					
12 AM					

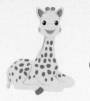

date : ....

	Feeding		Changing	Sleep	Notes
	Breast	Bottle			
12 AM					
1					
2					
3					
4					
5					
6					
7					
8					
9					
10					
11					
12 PM					
1					
2					
3					
4					
5					
6					
7					
8					
9					
10					
11					
12 AM					

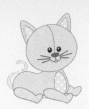

date : ....

	Feeding		Changing	Sleep	Notes
	Breast	Bottle			
12 AM					
1					
2					
3					
4					
5					
6					
7					
8					
9					
10					
11					
12 PM					
1					
2					
3					
4					
5					
6					
7					
8					
9					
10					
11					
12 AM					

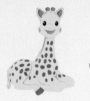

date : ....

	Feeding		Changing	Sleep	Notes
	Breast	Bottle			
12 AM					
1					
2					
3					
4					
5					
6					
7					
8					
9					
10					
11					
12 PM					
1					
2					
3					
4					
5					
6					
7					
8					
9					
10					
11					
12 AM					

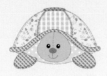

date : ....

	Feeding		Changing	Sleep	Notes
	Breast	Bottle			
12 AM					
1					
2					
3					
4					
5					
6					
7					
8					
9					
10					
11					
12 PM					
1					
2					
3					
4					
5					
6					
7					
8					
9					
10					
11					
12 AM					

date : ....

	Feeding		Changing	Sleep	Notes
	Breast	Bottle			
12 AM					
1					
2					
3					
4					
5					
6					
7					
8					
9					
10					
11					
12 PM					
1					
2					
3					
4					
5					
6					
7					
8					
9					
10					
11					
12 AM					

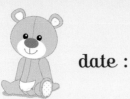

date : ....

	Feeding		Changing	Sleep	Notes
	Breast	Bottle			
12 AM					
1					
2					
3					
4					
5					
6					
7					
8					
9					
10					
11					
12 PM					
1					
2					
3					
4					
5					
6					
7					
8					
9					
10					
11					
12 AM					

date :

	Feeding		Changing	Sleep	Notes
	Breast	Bottle			
12 AM					
1					
2					
3					
4					
5					
6					
7					
8					
9					
10					
11					
12 PM					
1					
2					
3					
4					
5					
6					
7					
8					
9					
10					
11					
12 AM					

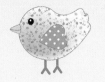

date : ....

	Feeding		Changing	Sleep	Notes
	Breast	Bottle			
12 AM					
1					
2					
3					
4					
5					
6					
7					
8					
9					
10					
11					
12 PM					
1					
2					
3					
4					
5					
6					
7					
8					
9					
10					
11					
12 AM					

date :

	Feeding		Changing	Sleep	Notes
	Breast	Bottle			
12 AM					
1					
2					
3					
4					
5					
6					
7					
8					
9					
10					
11					
12 PM					
1					
2					
3					
4					
5					
6					
7					
8					
9					
10					
11					
12 AM					

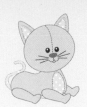

date : ....

	Feeding		Changing	Sleep	Notes
	Breast	Bottle			
12 AM	....	....	....	....	....
1	....	....	....	....	....
2	....	....	....	....	....
3	....	....	....	....	....
4	....	....	....	....	....
5	....	....	....	....	....
6	....	....	....	....	....
7	....	....	....	....	....
8	....	....	....	....	....
9	....	....	....	....	....
10	....	....	....	....	....
11	....	....	....	....	....
12 PM	....	....	....	....	....
1	....	....	....	....	....
2	....	....	....	....	....
3	....	....	....	....	....
4	....	....	....	....	....
5	....	....	....	....	....
6	....	....	....	....	....
7	....	....	....	....	....
8	....	....	....	....	....
9	....	....	....	....	....
10	....	....	....	....	....
11	....	....	....	....	....
12 AM	....	....	....	....	....

date : ....

	Feeding		Changing	Sleep	Notes
	Breast	Bottle			
12 AM					
1					
2					
3					
4					
5					
6					
7					
8					
9					
10					
11					
12 PM					
1					
2					
3					
4					
5					
6					
7					
8					
9					
10					
11					
12 AM					

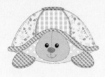

date : ....

	Feeding		Changing	Sleep	Notes
	Breast	Bottle			
12 AM					
1					
2					
3					
4					
5					
6					
7					
8					
9					
10					
11					
12 PM					
1					
2					
3					
4					
5					
6					
7					
8					
9					
10					
11					
12 AM					

date : ....

	Feeding		Changing	Sleep	Notes
	Breast	Bottle			
12 AM					
1					
2					
3					
4					
5					
6					
7					
8					
9					
10					
11					
12 PM					
1					
2					
3					
4					
5					
6					
7					
8					
9					
10					
11					
12 AM					

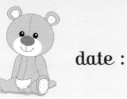

date : ....

	Feeding		Changing	Sleep	Notes
	Breast	Bottle			
12 AM					
1					
2					
3					
4					
5					
6					
7					
8					
9					
10					
11					
12 PM					
1					
2					
3					
4					
5					
6					
7					
8					
9					
10					
11					
12 AM					

date : ....

	Feeding		Changing	Sleep	Notes
	Breast	Bottle			
12 AM	....	....	....	....	....
1	....	....	....	....	....
2	....	....	....	....	....
3	....	....	....	....	....
4	....	....	....	....	....
5	....	....	....	....	....
6	....	....	....	....	....
7	....	....	....	....	....
8	....	....	....	....	....
9	....	....	....	....	....
10	....	....	....	....	....
11	....	....	....	....	....
12 PM	....	....	....	....	....
1	....	....	....	....	....
2	....	....	....	....	....
3	....	....	....	....	....
4	....	....	....	....	....
5	....	....	....	....	....
6	....	....	....	....	....
7	....	....	....	....	....
8	....	....	....	....	....
9	....	....	....	....	....
10	....	....	....	....	....
11	....	....	....	....	....
12 AM	....	....	....	....	....

date : ....

	Feeding		Changing	Sleep	Notes
	Breast	Bottle			
12 AM					
1					
2					
3					
4					
5					
6					
7					
8					
9					
10					
11					
12 PM					
1					
2					
3					
4					
5					
6					
7					
8					
9					
10					
11					
12 AM					

date : ....

	Feeding		Changing	Sleep	Notes
	Breast	Bottle			
12 AM					
1					
2					
3					
4					
5					
6					
7					
8					
9					
10					
11					
12 PM					
1					
2					
3					
4					
5					
6					
7					
8					
9					
10					
11					
12 AM					

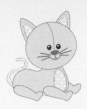

date :

	Feeding		Changing	Sleep	Notes
	Breast	Bottle			
12 AM					
1					
2					
3					
4					
5					
6					
7					
8					
9					
10					
11					
12 PM					
1					
2					
3					
4					
5					
6					
7					
8					
9					
10					
11					
12 AM					

date : ....

	Feeding		Changing	Sleep	Notes
	Breast	Bottle			
12 AM					
1					
2					
3					
4					
5					
6					
7					
8					
9					
10					
11					
12 PM					
1					
2					
3					
4					
5					
6					
7					
8					
9					
10					
11					
12 AM					

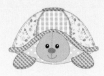

date : ....

	Feeding		Changing	Sleep	Notes
	Breast	Bottle			
12 AM	....	....	....	....	....
1	....	....	....	....	....
2	....	....	....	....	....
3	....	....	....	....	....
4	....	....	....	....	....
5	....	....	....	....	....
6	....	....	....	....	....
7	....	....	....	....	....
8	....	....	....	....	....
9	....	....	....	....	....
10	....	....	....	....	....
11	....	....	....	....	....
12 PM	....	....	....	....	....
1	....	....	....	....	....
2	....	....	....	....	....
3	....	....	....	....	....
4	....	....	....	....	....
5	....	....	....	....	....
6	....	....	....	....	....
7	....	....	....	....	....
8	....	....	....	....	....
9	....	....	....	....	....
10	....	....	....	....	....
11	....	....	....	....	....
12 AM	....	....	....	....	....

date :

	Feeding		Changing	Sleep	Notes
	Breast	Bottle			
12 AM					
1					
2					
3					
4					
5					
6					
7					
8					
9					
10					
11					
12 PM					
1					
2					
3					
4					
5					
6					
7					
8					
9					
10					
11					
12 AM					

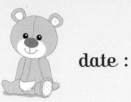

date : ....

	Feeding		Changing	Sleep	Notes
	Breast	Bottle			
12 AM					
1					
2					
3					
4					
5					
6					
7					
8					
9					
10					
11					
12 PM					
1					
2					
3					
4					
5					
6					
7					
8					
9					
10					
11					
12 AM					

date : ....

	Feeding		Changing	Sleep	Notes
	Breast	Bottle			
12 AM					
1					
2					
3					
4					
5					
6					
7					
8					
9					
10					
11					
12 PM					
1					
2					
3					
4					
5					
6					
7					
8					
9					
10					
11					
12 AM					

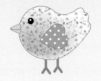

date : ....

	Feeding		Changing	Sleep	Notes
	Breast	Bottle			
12 AM					
1					
2					
3					
4					
5					
6					
7					
8					
9					
10					
11					
12 PM					
1					
2					
3					
4					
5					
6					
7					
8					
9					
10					
11					
12 AM					

date : ....

	Feeding		Changing	Sleep	Notes
	Breast	Bottle			
12 AM	....	....	....	....	....
1	....	....	....	....	....
2	....	....	....	....	....
3	....	....	....	....	....
4	....	....	....	....	....
5	....	....	....	....	....
6	....	....	....	....	....
7	....	....	....	....	....
8	....	....	....	....	....
9	....	....	....	....	....
10	....	....	....	....	....
11	....	....	....	....	....
12 PM	....	....	....	....	....
1	....	....	....	....	....
2	....	....	....	....	....
3	....	....	....	....	....
4	....	....	....	....	....
5	....	....	....	....	....
6	....	....	....	....	....
7	....	....	....	....	....
8	....	....	....	....	....
9	....	....	....	....	....
10	....	....	....	....	....
11	....	....	....	....	....
12 AM	....	....	....	....	....

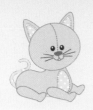

date : ....

	Feeding		Changing	Sleep	Notes
	Breast	Bottle			
12 AM					
1					
2					
3					
4					
5					
6					
7					
8					
9					
10					
11					
12 PM					
1					
2					
3					
4					
5					
6					
7					
8					
9					
10					
11					
12 AM					

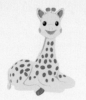

date : ....

	Feeding		Changing	Sleep	Notes
	Breast	Bottle			
12 AM					
1					
2					
3					
4					
5					
6					
7					
8					
9					
10					
11					
12 PM					
1					
2					
3					
4					
5					
6					
7					
8					
9					
10					
11					
12 AM					

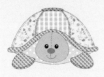

date : ....

	Feeding		Changing	Sleep	Notes
	Breast	Bottle			
12 AM					
1					
2					
3					
4					
5					
6					
7					
8					
9					
10					
11					
12 PM					
1					
2					
3					
4					
5					
6					
7					
8					
9					
10					
11					
12 AM					

date : ....

	Feeding		Changing	Sleep	Notes
	Breast	Bottle			
12 AM					
1					
2					
3					
4					
5					
6					
7					
8					
9					
10					
11					
12 PM					
1					
2					
3					
4					
5					
6					
7					
8					
9					
10					
11					
12 AM					

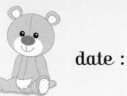

date :

	Feeding		Changing	Sleep	Notes
	Breast	Bottle			
12 AM					
1					
2					
3					
4					
5					
6					
7					
8					
9					
10					
11					
12 PM					
1					
2					
3					
4					
5					
6					
7					
8					
9					
10					
11					
12 AM					

date : ....

	Feeding		Changing	Sleep	Notes
	Breast	Bottle			
12 AM					
1					
2					
3					
4					
5					
6					
7					
8					
9					
10					
11					
12 PM					
1					
2					
3					
4					
5					
6					
7					
8					
9					
10					
11					
12 AM					

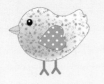

date : ....

	Feeding		Changing	Sleep	Notes
	Breast	Bottle			
12 AM					
1					
2					
3					
4					
5					
6					
7					
8					
9					
10					
11					
12 PM					
1					
2					
3					
4					
5					
6					
7					
8					
9					
10					
11					
12 AM					

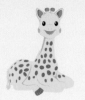

date : ....

	Feeding		Changing	Sleep	Notes
	Breast	Bottle			
12 AM					
1					
2					
3					
4					
5					
6					
7					
8					
9					
10					
11					
12 PM					
1					
2					
3					
4					
5					
6					
7					
8					
9					
10					
11					
12 AM					

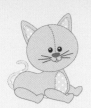

date : ....

	Feeding		Changing	Sleep	Notes
	Breast	Bottle			
12 AM					
1					
2					
3					
4					
5					
6					
7					
8					
9					
10					
11					
12 PM					
1					
2					
3					
4					
5					
6					
7					
8					
9					
10					
11					
12 AM					

date : ....

	Feeding		Changing	Sleep	Notes
	Breast	Bottle			
12 AM	....	....	....	....	....
1	....	....	....	....	....
2	....	....	....	....	....
3	....	....	....	....	....
4	....	....	....	....	....
5	....	....	....	....	....
6	....	....	....	....	....
7	....	....	....	....	....
8	....	....	....	....	....
9	....	....	....	....	....
10	....	....	....	....	....
11	....	....	....	....	....
12 PM	....	....	....	....	....
1	....	....	....	....	....
2	....	....	....	....	....
3	....	....	....	....	....
4	....	....	....	....	....
5	....	....	....	....	....
6	....	....	....	....	....
7	....	....	....	....	....
8	....	....	....	....	....
9	....	....	....	....	....
10	....	....	....	....	....
11	....	....	....	....	....
12 AM	....	....	....	....	....

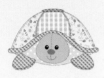

date : ....

	Feeding		Changing	Sleep	Notes
	Breast	Bottle			
12 AM	....	....	....	....	....
1	....	....	....	....	....
2	....	....	....	....	....
3	....	....	....	....	....
4	....	....	....	....	....
5	....	....	....	....	....
6	....	....	....	....	....
7	....	....	....	....	....
8	....	....	....	....	....
9	....	....	....	....	....
10	....	....	....	....	....
11	....	....	....	....	....
12 PM	....	....	....	....	....
1	....	....	....	....	....
2	....	....	....	....	....
3	....	....	....	....	....
4	....	....	....	....	....
5	....	....	....	....	....
6	....	....	....	....	....
7	....	....	....	....	....
8	....	....	....	....	....
9	....	....	....	....	....
10	....	....	....	....	....
11	....	....	....	....	....
12 AM	....	....	....	....	....

date : ....

	Feeding		Changing	Sleep	Notes
	Breast	Bottle			
12 AM					
1					
2					
3					
4					
5					
6					
7					
8					
9					
10					
11					
12 PM					
1					
2					
3					
4					
5					
6					
7					
8					
9					
10					
11					
12 AM					

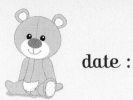

date : ....

	Feeding		Changing	Sleep	Notes
	Breast	Bottle			
12 AM					
1					
2					
3					
4					
5					
6					
7					
8					
9					
10					
11					
12 PM					
1					
2					
3					
4					
5					
6					
7					
8					
9					
10					
11					
12 AM					

date : ....

	Feeding		Changing	Sleep	Notes
	Breast	Bottle			
12 AM	....	....	....	....	....
1	....	....	....	....	....
2	....	....	....	....	....
3	....	....	....	....	....
4	....	....	....	....	....
5	....	....	....	....	....
6	....	....	....	....	....
7	....	....	....	....	....
8	....	....	....	....	....
9	....	....	....	....	....
10	....	....	....	....	....
11	....	....	....	....	....
12 PM	....	....	....	....	....
1	....	....	....	....	....
2	....	....	....	....	....
3	....	....	....	....	....
4	....	....	....	....	....
5	....	....	....	....	....
6	....	....	....	....	....
7	....	....	....	....	....
8	....	....	....	....	....
9	....	....	....	....	....
10	....	....	....	....	....
11	....	....	....	....	....
12 AM	....	....	....	....	....

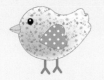

date :

	Feeding		Changing	Sleep	Notes
	Breast	Bottle			
12 AM					
1					
2					
3					
4					
5					
6					
7					
8					
9					
10					
11					
12 PM					
1					
2					
3					
4					
5					
6					
7					
8					
9					
10					
11					
12 AM					

date : ....

	Feeding		Changing	Sleep	Notes
	Breast	Bottle			
12 AM					
1					
2					
3					
4					
5					
6					
7					
8					
9					
10					
11					
12 PM					
1					
2					
3					
4					
5					
6					
7					
8					
9					
10					
11					
12 AM					

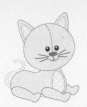

date : ....

	Feeding		Changing	Sleep	Notes
	Breast	Bottle			
12 AM					
1					
2					
3					
4					
5					
6					
7					
8					
9					
10					
11					
12 PM					
1					
2					
3					
4					
5					
6					
7					
8					
9					
10					
11					
12 AM					

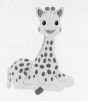

date : ....

	Feeding		Changing	Sleep	Notes
	Breast	Bottle			
12 AM					
1					
2					
3					
4					
5					
6					
7					
8					
9					
10					
11					
12 PM					
1					
2					
3					
4					
5					
6					
7					
8					
9					
10					
11					
12 AM					

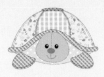

date : ....

	Feeding		Changing	Sleep	Notes
	Breast	Bottle			
12 AM	....	....	....	....	....
1	....	....	....	....	....
2	....	....	....	....	....
3	....	....	....	....	....
4	....	....	....	....	....
5	....	....	....	....	....
6	....	....	....	....	....
7	....	....	....	....	....
8	....	....	....	....	....
9	....	....	....	....	....
10	....	....	....	....	....
11	....	....	....	....	....
12 PM	....	....	....	....	....
1	....	....	....	....	....
2	....	....	....	....	....
3	....	....	....	....	....
4	....	....	....	....	....
5	....	....	....	....	....
6	....	....	....	....	....
7	....	....	....	....	....
8	....	....	....	....	....
9	....	....	....	....	....
10	....	....	....	....	....
11	....	....	....	....	....
12 AM	....	....	....	....	....

date : ....

	Feeding		Changing	Sleep	Notes
	Breast	Bottle			
12 AM					
1					
2					
3					
4					
5					
6					
7					
8					
9					
10					
11					
12 PM					
1					
2					
3					
4					
5					
6					
7					
8					
9					
10					
11					
12 AM					

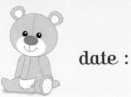

date : ....

	Feeding		Changing	Sleep	Notes
	Breast	Bottle			
12 AM					
1					
2					
3					
4					
5					
6					
7					
8					
9					
10					
11					
12 PM					
1					
2					
3					
4					
5					
6					
7					
8					
9					
10					
11					
12 AM					

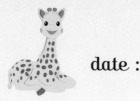

date : ....

	Feeding		Changing	Sleep	Notes
	Breast	Bottle			
12 AM	....	....	....	....	....
1	....	....	....	....	....
2	....	....	....	....	....
3	....	....	....	....	....
4	....	....	....	....	....
5	....	....	....	....	....
6	....	....	....	....	....
7	....	....	....	....	....
8	....	....	....	....	....
9	....	....	....	....	....
10	....	....	....	....	....
11	....	....	....	....	....
12 PM	....	....	....	....	....
1	....	....	....	....	....
2	....	....	....	....	....
3	....	....	....	....	....
4	....	....	....	....	....
5	....	....	....	....	....
6	....	....	....	....	....
7	....	....	....	....	....
8	....	....	....	....	....
9	....	....	....	....	....
10	....	....	....	....	....
11	....	....	....	....	....
12 AM	....	....	....	....	....

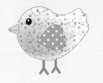

date : ....

	Feeding		Changing	Sleep	Notes
	Breast	Bottle			
12 AM					
1					
2					
3					
4					
5					
6					
7					
8					
9					
10					
11					
12 PM					
1					
2					
3					
4					
5					
6					
7					
8					
9					
10					
11					
12 AM					

date : ....

	Feeding		Changing	Sleep	Notes
	Breast	Bottle			
12 AM					
1					
2					
3					
4					
5					
6					
7					
8					
9					
10					
11					
12 PM					
1					
2					
3					
4					
5					
6					
7					
8					
9					
10					
11					
12 AM					

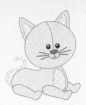

date : ....

	Feeding		Changing	Sleep	Notes
	Breast	Bottle			
12 AM					
1					
2					
3					
4					
5					
6					
7					
8					
9					
10					
11					
12 PM					
1					
2					
3					
4					
5					
6					
7					
8					
9					
10					
11					
12 AM					

date :

	Feeding		Changing	Sleep	Notes
	Breast	Bottle			
12 AM					
1					
2					
3					
4					
5					
6					
7					
8					
9					
10					
11					
12 PM					
1					
2					
3					
4					
5					
6					
7					
8					
9					
10					
11					
12 AM					

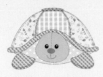

date : ....

	Feeding		Changing	Sleep	Notes
	Breast	Bottle			
12 AM	....	....	....	....	....
1	....	....	....	....	....
2	....	....	....	....	....
3	....	....	....	....	....
4	....	....	....	....	....
5	....	....	....	....	....
6	....	....	....	....	....
7	....	....	....	....	....
8	....	....	....	....	....
9	....	....	....	....	....
10	....	....	....	....	....
11	....	....	....	....	....
12 PM	....	....	....	....	....
1	....	....	....	....	....
2	....	....	....	....	....
3	....	....	....	....	....
4	....	....	....	....	....
5	....	....	....	....	....
6	....	....	....	....	....
7	....	....	....	....	....
8	....	....	....	....	....
9	....	....	....	....	....
10	....	....	....	....	....
11	....	....	....	....	....
12 AM	....	....	....	....	....

date : ....

	Feeding		Changing	Sleep	Notes
	Breast	Bottle			
12 AM	....	....	....	....	....
1	....	....	....	....	....
2	....	....	....	....	....
3	....	....	....	....	....
4	....	....	....	....	....
5	....	....	....	....	....
6	....	....	....	....	....
7	....	....	....	....	....
8	....	....	....	....	....
9	....	....	....	....	....
10	....	....	....	....	....
11	....	....	....	....	....
12 PM	....	....	....	....	....
1	....	....	....	....	....
2	....	....	....	....	....
3	....	....	....	....	....
4	....	....	....	....	....
5	....	....	....	....	....
6	....	....	....	....	....
7	....	....	....	....	....
8	....	....	....	....	....
9	....	....	....	....	....
10	....	....	....	....	....
11	....	....	....	....	....
12 AM	....	....	....	....	....

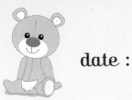

date : ....

	Feeding		Changing	Sleep	Notes
	Breast	Bottle			
12 AM					
1					
2					
3					
4					
5					
6					
7					
8					
9					
10					
11					
12 PM					
1					
2					
3					
4					
5					
6					
7					
8					
9					
10					
11					
12 AM					

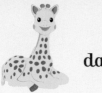

date :

	Feeding		Changing	Sleep	Notes
	Breast	Bottle			
12 AM					
1					
2					
3					
4					
5					
6					
7					
8					
9					
10					
11					
12 PM					
1					
2					
3					
4					
5					
6					
7					
8					
9					
10					
11					
12 AM					

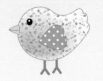

date : ....

	Feeding		Changing	Sleep	Notes
	Breast	Bottle			
12 AM	....	....	....	....	....
1	....	....	....	....	....
2	....	....	....	....	....
3	....	....	....	....	....
4	....	....	....	....	....
5	....	....	....	....	....
6	....	....	....	....	....
7	....	....	....	....	....
8	....	....	....	....	....
9	....	....	....	....	....
10	....	....	....	....	....
11	....	....	....	....	....
12 PM	....	....	....	....	....
1	....	....	....	....	....
2	....	....	....	....	....
3	....	....	....	....	....
4	....	....	....	....	....
5	....	....	....	....	....
6	....	....	....	....	....
7	....	....	....	....	....
8	....	....	....	....	....
9	....	....	....	....	....
10	....	....	....	....	....
11	....	....	....	....	....
12 AM	....	....	....	....	....

date : ....

	Feeding		Changing	Sleep	Notes
	Breast	Bottle			
12 AM					
1					
2					
3					
4					
5					
6					
7					
8					
9					
10					
11					
12 PM					
1					
2					
3					
4					
5					
6					
7					
8					
9					
10					
11					
12 AM					

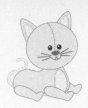

date :

	Feeding		Changing	Sleep	Notes
	Breast	Bottle			
12 AM					
1					
2					
3					
4					
5					
6					
7					
8					
9					
10					
11					
12 PM					
1					
2					
3					
4					
5					
6					
7					
8					
9					
10					
11					
12 AM					

date : ....

	Feeding		Changing	Sleep	Notes
	Breast	Bottle			
12 AM					
1					
2					
3					
4					
5					
6					
7					
8					
9					
10					
11					
12 PM					
1					
2					
3					
4					
5					
6					
7					
8					
9					
10					
11					
12 AM					

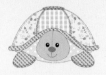

date : ....

	Feeding		Changing	Sleep	Notes
	Breast	Bottle			
12 AM					
1					
2					
3					
4					
5					
6					
7					
8					
9					
10					
11					
12 PM					
1					
2					
3					
4					
5					
6					
7					
8					
9					
10					
11					
12 AM					

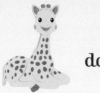

date : ....

	Feeding		Changing	Sleep	Notes
	Breast	Bottle			
12 AM	....	....	....	....	....
1	....	....	....	....	....
2	....	....	....	....	....
3	....	....	....	....	....
4	....	....	....	....	....
5	....	....	....	....	....
6	....	....	....	....	....
7	....	....	....	....	....
8	....	....	....	....	....
9	....	....	....	....	....
10	....	....	....	....	....
11	....	....	....	....	....
12 PM	....	....	....	....	....
1	....	....	....	....	....
2	....	....	....	....	....
3	....	....	....	....	....
4	....	....	....	....	....
5	....	....	....	....	....
6	....	....	....	....	....
7	....	....	....	....	....
8	....	....	....	....	....
9	....	....	....	....	....
10	....	....	....	....	....
11	....	....	....	....	....
12 AM	....	....	....	....	....

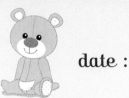

date : ....

	Feeding		Changing	Sleep	Notes
	Breast	Bottle			
12 AM					
1					
2					
3					
4					
5					
6					
7					
8					
9					
10					
11					
12 PM					
1					
2					
3					
4					
5					
6					
7					
8					
9					
10					
11					
12 AM					

date : ....

	Feeding		Changing	Sleep	Notes
	Breast	Bottle			
12 AM					
1					
2					
3					
4					
5					
6					
7					
8					
9					
10					
11					
12 PM					
1					
2					
3					
4					
5					
6					
7					
8					
9					
10					
11					
12 AM					

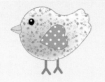

date : ....

	Feeding		Changing	Sleep	Notes
	Breast	Bottle			
12 AM					
1					
2					
3					
4					
5					
6					
7					
8					
9					
10					
11					
12 PM					
1					
2					
3					
4					
5					
6					
7					
8					
9					
10					
11					
12 AM					

date : ....

	Feeding		Changing	Sleep	Notes
	Breast	Bottle			
12 AM					
1					
2					
3					
4					
5					
6					
7					
8					
9					
10					
11					
12 PM					
1					
2					
3					
4					
5					
6					
7					
8					
9					
10					
11					
12 AM					

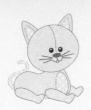

date :

	Feeding		Changing	Sleep	Notes
	Breast	Bottle			
12 AM					
1					
2					
3					
4					
5					
6					
7					
8					
9					
10					
11					
12 PM					
1					
2					
3					
4					
5					
6					
7					
8					
9					
10					
11					
12 AM					

date : ....

	Feeding		Changing	Sleep	Notes
	Breast	Bottle			
12 AM					
1					
2					
3					
4					
5					
6					
7					
8					
9					
10					
11					
12 PM					
1					
2					
3					
4					
5					
6					
7					
8					
9					
10					
11					
12 AM					

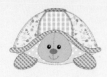

date : ....

	Feeding		Changing	Sleep	Notes
	Breast	Bottle			
12 AM	....	....	....	....	....
1	....	....	....	....	....
2	....	....	....	....	....
3	....	....	....	....	....
4	....	....	....	....	....
5	....	....	....	....	....
6	....	....	....	....	....
7	....	....	....	....	....
8	....	....	....	....	....
9	....	....	....	....	....
10	....	....	....	....	....
11	....	....	....	....	....
12 PM	....	....	....	....	....
1	....	....	....	....	....
2	....	....	....	....	....
3	....	....	....	....	....
4	....	....	....	....	....
5	....	....	....	....	....
6	....	....	....	....	....
7	....	....	....	....	....
8	....	....	....	....	....
9	....	....	....	....	....
10	....	....	....	....	....
11	....	....	....	....	....
12 AM	....	....	....	....	....

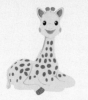

date : ....

	Feeding		Changing	Sleep	Notes
	Breast	Bottle			
12 AM					
1					
2					
3					
4					
5					
6					
7					
8					
9					
10					
11					
12 PM					
1					
2					
3					
4					
5					
6					
7					
8					
9					
10					
11					
12 AM					

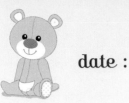

date :

	Feeding		Changing	Sleep	Notes
	Breast	Bottle			
12 AM					
1					
2					
3					
4					
5					
6					
7					
8					
9					
10					
11					
12 PM					
1					
2					
3					
4					
5					
6					
7					
8					
9					
10					
11					
12 AM					

date : ....

	Feeding		Changing	Sleep	Notes
	Breast	Bottle			
12 AM	....	....	....	....	....
1	....	....	....	....	....
2	....	....	....	....	....
3	....	....	....	....	....
4	....	....	....	....	....
5	....	....	....	....	....
6	....	....	....	....	....
7	....	....	....	....	....
8	....	....	....	....	....
9	....	....	....	....	....
10	....	....	....	....	....
11	....	....	....	....	....
12 PM	....	....	....	....	....
1	....	....	....	....	....
2	....	....	....	....	....
3	....	....	....	....	....
4	....	....	....	....	....
5	....	....	....	....	....
6	....	....	....	....	....
7	....	....	....	....	....
8	....	....	....	....	....
9	....	....	....	....	....
10	....	....	....	....	....
11	....	....	....	....	....
12 AM	....	....	....	....	....

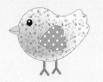

date : ....

	Feeding		Changing	Sleep	Notes
	Breast	Bottle			
12 AM					
1					
2					
3					
4					
5					
6					
7					
8					
9					
10					
11					
12 PM					
1					
2					
3					
4					
5					
6					
7					
8					
9					
10					
11					
12 AM					

date :

	Feeding		Changing	Sleep	Notes
	Breast	Bottle			
12 AM					
1					
2					
3					
4					
5					
6					
7					
8					
9					
10					
11					
12 PM					
1					
2					
3					
4					
5					
6					
7					
8					
9					
10					
11					
12 AM					

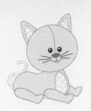

date : ....

	Feeding		Changing	Sleep	Notes
	Breast	Bottle			
12 AM					
1					
2					
3					
4					
5					
6					
7					
8					
9					
10					
11					
12 PM					
1					
2					
3					
4					
5					
6					
7					
8					
9					
10					
11					
12 AM					

date : ....

	Feeding		Changing	Sleep	Notes
	Breast	Bottle			
12 AM					
1					
2					
3					
4					
5					
6					
7					
8					
9					
10					
11					
12 PM					
1					
2					
3					
4					
5					
6					
7					
8					
9					
10					
11					
12 AM					

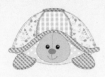

date : ....

	Feeding		Changing	Sleep	Notes
	Breast	Bottle			
12 AM					
1					
2					
3					
4					
5					
6					
7					
8					
9					
10					
11					
12 PM					
1					
2					
3					
4					
5					
6					
7					
8					
9					
10					
11					
12 AM					

date : ....

	Feeding		Changing	Sleep	Notes
	Breast	Bottle			
12 AM					
1					
2					
3					
4					
5					
6					
7					
8					
9					
10					
11					
12 PM					
1					
2					
3					
4					
5					
6					
7					
8					
9					
10					
11					
12 AM					

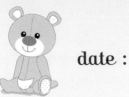

date : ....

	Feeding		Changing	Sleep	Notes
	Breast	Bottle			
12 AM	....	....	....	....	....
1	....	....	....	....	....
2	....	....	....	....	....
3	....	....	....	....	....
4	....	....	....	....	....
5	....	....	....	....	....
6	....	....	....	....	....
7	....	....	....	....	....
8	....	....	....	....	....
9	....	....	....	....	....
10	....	....	....	....	....
11	....	....	....	....	....
12 PM	....	....	....	....	....
1	....	....	....	....	....
2	....	....	....	....	....
3	....	....	....	....	....
4	....	....	....	....	....
5	....	....	....	....	....
6	....	....	....	....	....
7	....	....	....	....	....
8	....	....	....	....	....
9	....	....	....	....	....
10	....	....	....	....	....
11	....	....	....	....	....
12 AM	....	....	....	....	....

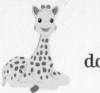

date : ....

	Feeding		Changing	Sleep	Notes
	Breast	Bottle			
12 AM					
1					
2					
3					
4					
5					
6					
7					
8					
9					
10					
11					
12 PM					
1					
2					
3					
4					
5					
6					
7					
8					
9					
10					
11					
12 AM					

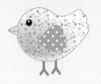

date : ....

	Feeding		Changing	Sleep	Notes
	Breast	Bottle			
12 AM					
1					
2					
3					
4					
5					
6					
7					
8					
9					
10					
11					
12 PM					
1					
2					
3					
4					
5					
6					
7					
8					
9					
10					
11					
12 AM					

date : ....

	Feeding		Changing	Sleep	Notes
	Breast	Bottle			
12 AM					
1					
2					
3					
4					
5					
6					
7					
8					
9					
10					
11					
12 PM					
1					
2					
3					
4					
5					
6					
7					
8					
9					
10					
11					
12 AM					

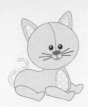

date : ....

	Feeding		Changing	Sleep	Notes
	Breast	Bottle			
12 AM					
1					
2					
3					
4					
5					
6					
7					
8					
9					
10					
11					
12 PM					
1					
2					
3					
4					
5					
6					
7					
8					
9					
10					
11					
12 AM					

date : ....

	Feeding		Changing	Sleep	Notes
	Breast	Bottle			
12 AM					
1					
2					
3					
4					
5					
6					
7					
8					
9					
10					
11					
12 PM					
1					
2					
3					
4					
5					
6					
7					
8					
9					
10					
11					
12 AM					

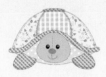

date : ....

	Feeding		Changing	Sleep	Notes
	Breast	Bottle			
12 AM					
1					
2					
3					
4					
5					
6					
7					
8					
9					
10					
11					
12 PM					
1					
2					
3					
4					
5					
6					
7					
8					
9					
10					
11					
12 AM					

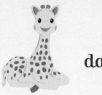

date : ....

	Feeding		Changing	Sleep	Notes
	Breast	Bottle			
12 AM	....	....	....	....	....
1	....	....	....	....	....
2	....	....	....	....	....
3	....	....	....	....	....
4	....	....	....	....	....
5	....	....	....	....	....
6	....	....	....	....	....
7	....	....	....	....	....
8	....	....	....	....	....
9	....	....	....	....	....
10	....	....	....	....	....
11	....	....	....	....	....
12 PM	....	....	....	....	....
1	....	....	....	....	....
2	....	....	....	....	....
3	....	....	....	....	....
4	....	....	....	....	....
5	....	....	....	....	....
6	....	....	....	....	....
7	....	....	....	....	....
8	....	....	....	....	....
9	....	....	....	....	....
10	....	....	....	....	....
11	....	....	....	....	....
12 AM	....	....	....	....	....

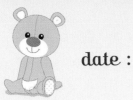

date : ....

	Feeding		Changing	Sleep	Notes
	Breast	Bottle			
12 AM	....	....	....	....	....
1	....	....	....	....	....
2	....	....	....	....	....
3	....	....	....	....	....
4	....	....	....	....	....
5	....	....	....	....	....
6	....	....	....	....	....
7	....	....	....	....	....
8	....	....	....	....	....
9	....	....	....	....	....
10	....	....	....	....	....
11	....	....	....	....	....
12 PM	....	....	....	....	....
1	....	....	....	....	....
2	....	....	....	....	....
3	....	....	....	....	....
4	....	....	....	....	....
5	....	....	....	....	....
6	....	....	....	....	....
7	....	....	....	....	....
8	....	....	....	....	....
9	....	....	....	....	....
10	....	....	....	....	....
11	....	....	....	....	....
12 AM	....	....	....	....	....

date : ....

	Feeding		Changing	Sleep	Notes
	Breast	Bottle			
12 AM					
1					
2					
3					
4					
5					
6					
7					
8					
9					
10					
11					
12 PM					
1					
2					
3					
4					
5					
6					
7					
8					
9					
10					
11					
12 AM					

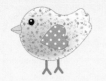

date : ....

	Feeding		Changing	Sleep	Notes
	Breast	Bottle			
12 AM					
1					
2					
3					
4					
5					
6					
7					
8					
9					
10					
11					
12 PM					
1					
2					
3					
4					
5					
6					
7					
8					
9					
10					
11					
12 AM					

date : ....

	Feeding		Changing	Sleep	Notes
	Breast	Bottle			
12 AM					
1					
2					
3					
4					
5					
6					
7					
8					
9					
10					
11					
12 PM					
1					
2					
3					
4					
5					
6					
7					
8					
9					
10					
11					
12 AM					

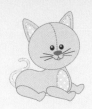

date : ....

	Feeding		Changing	Sleep	Notes
	Breast	Bottle			
12 AM					
1					
2					
3					
4					
5					
6					
7					
8					
9					
10					
11					
12 PM					
1					
2					
3					
4					
5					
6					
7					
8					
9					
10					
11					
12 AM					

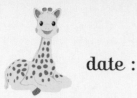

date : ....

	Feeding		Changing	Sleep	Notes
	Breast	Bottle			
12 AM					
1					
2					
3					
4					
5					
6					
7					
8					
9					
10					
11					
12 PM					
1					
2					
3					
4					
5					
6					
7					
8					
9					
10					
11					
12 AM					

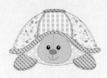

date : ....

	Feeding		Changing	Sleep	Notes
	Breast	Bottle			
12 AM					
1					
2					
3					
4					
5					
6					
7					
8					
9					
10					
11					
12 PM					
1					
2					
3					
4					
5					
6					
7					
8					
9					
10					
11					
12 AM					

date : ....

	Feeding		Changing	Sleep	Notes
	Breast	Bottle			
12 AM					
1					
2					
3					
4					
5					
6					
7					
8					
9					
10					
11					
12 PM					
1					
2					
3					
4					
5					
6					
7					
8					
9					
10					
11					
12 AM					

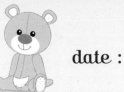

date : ....

	Feeding		Changing	Sleep	Notes
	Breast	Bottle			
12 AM					
1					
2					
3					
4					
5					
6					
7					
8					
9					
10					
11					
12 PM					
1					
2					
3					
4					
5					
6					
7					
8					
9					
10					
11					
12 AM					

date : ....

	Feeding		Changing	Sleep	Notes
	Breast	Bottle			
12 AM					
1					
2					
3					
4					
5					
6					
7					
8					
9					
10					
11					
12 PM					
1					
2					
3					
4					
5					
6					
7					
8					
9					
10					
11					
12 AM					

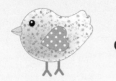

date : ....

	Feeding		Changing	Sleep	Notes
	Breast	Bottle			
12 AM					
1					
2					
3					
4					
5					
6					
7					
8					
9					
10					
11					
12 PM					
1					
2					
3					
4					
5					
6					
7					
8					
9					
10					
11					
12 AM					

date : ....

	Feeding		Changing	Sleep	Notes
	Breast	Bottle			
12 AM	....	....	....	....	....
1	....	....	....	....	....
2	....	....	....	....	....
3	....	....	....	....	....
4	....	....	....	....	....
5	....	....	....	....	....
6	....	....	....	....	....
7	....	....	....	....	....
8	....	....	....	....	....
9	....	....	....	....	....
10	....	....	....	....	....
11	....	....	....	....	....
12 PM	....	....	....	....	....
1	....	....	....	....	....
2	....	....	....	....	....
3	....	....	....	....	....
4	....	....	....	....	....
5	....	....	....	....	....
6	....	....	....	....	....
7	....	....	....	....	....
8	....	....	....	....	....
9	....	....	....	....	....
10	....	....	....	....	....
11	....	....	....	....	....
12 AM	....	....	....	....	....

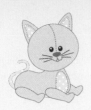

date : ....

	Feeding		Changing	Sleep	Notes
	Breast	Bottle			
12 AM					
1					
2					
3					
4					
5					
6					
7					
8					
9					
10					
11					
12 PM					
1					
2					
3					
4					
5					
6					
7					
8					
9					
10					
11					
12 AM					

date : ....

	Feeding		Changing	Sleep	Notes
	Breast	Bottle			
12 AM					
1					
2					
3					
4					
5					
6					
7					
8					
9					
10					
11					
12 PM					
1					
2					
3					
4					
5					
6					
7					
8					
9					
10					
11					
12 AM					

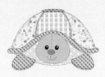

date : ....

	Feeding		Changing	Sleep	Notes
	Breast	Bottle			
12 AM	....	....	....	....	....
1	....	....	....	....	....
2	....	....	....	....	....
3	....	....	....	....	....
4	....	....	....	....	....
5	....	....	....	....	....
6	....	....	....	....	....
7	....	....	....	....	....
8	....	....	....	....	....
9	....	....	....	....	....
10	....	....	....	....	....
11	....	....	....	....	....
12 PM	....	....	....	....	....
1	....	....	....	....	....
2	....	....	....	....	....
3	....	....	....	....	....
4	....	....	....	....	....
5	....	....	....	....	....
6	....	....	....	....	....
7	....	....	....	....	....
8	....	....	....	....	....
9	....	....	....	....	....
10	....	....	....	....	....
11	....	....	....	....	....
12 AM	....	....	....	....	....

date : ....

	Feeding		Changing	Sleep	Notes
	Breast	Bottle			
12 AM					
1					
2					
3					
4					
5					
6					
7					
8					
9					
10					
11					
12 PM					
1					
2					
3					
4					
5					
6					
7					
8					
9					
10					
11					
12 AM					

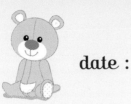

date : ....

	Feeding		Changing	Sleep	Notes
	Breast	Bottle			
12 AM					
1					
2					
3					
4					
5					
6					
7					
8					
9					
10					
11					
12 PM					
1					
2					
3					
4					
5					
6					
7					
8					
9					
10					
11					
12 AM					

date :

	Feeding		Changing	Sleep	Notes
	Breast	Bottle			
12 AM					
1					
2					
3					
4					
5					
6					
7					
8					
9					
10					
11					
12 PM					
1					
2					
3					
4					
5					
6					
7					
8					
9					
10					
11					
12 AM					

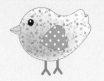

date : ....

	Feeding		Changing	Sleep	Notes
	Breast	Bottle			
12 AM					
1					
2					
3					
4					
5					
6					
7					
8					
9					
10					
11					
12 PM					
1					
2					
3					
4					
5					
6					
7					
8					
9					
10					
11					
12 AM					

date : ....

	Feeding		Changing	Sleep	Notes
	Breast	Bottle			
12 AM					
1					
2					
3					
4					
5					
6					
7					
8					
9					
10					
11					
12 PM					
1					
2					
3					
4					
5					
6					
7					
8					
9					
10					
11					
12 AM					

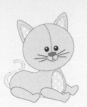

date : ....

	Feeding		Changing	Sleep	Notes
	Breast	Bottle			
12 AM	....	....	....	....	....
1	....	....	....	....	....
2	....	....	....	....	....
3	....	....	....	....	....
4	....	....	....	....	....
5	....	....	....	....	....
6	....	....	....	....	....
7	....	....	....	....	....
8	....	....	....	....	....
9	....	....	....	....	....
10	....	....	....	....	....
11	....	....	....	....	....
12 PM	....	....	....	....	....
1	....	....	....	....	....
2	....	....	....	....	....
3	....	....	....	....	....
4	....	....	....	....	....
5	....	....	....	....	....
6	....	....	....	....	....
7	....	....	....	....	....
8	....	....	....	....	....
9	....	....	....	....	....
10	....	....	....	....	....
11	....	....	....	....	....
12 AM	....	....	....	....	....

date : ....

	Feeding		Changing	Sleep	Notes
	Breast	Bottle			
12 AM					
1					
2					
3					
4					
5					
6					
7					
8					
9					
10					
11					
12 PM					
1					
2					
3					
4					
5					
6					
7					
8					
9					
10					
11					
12 AM					

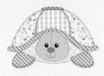

date : ....

	Feeding		Changing	Sleep	Notes
	Breast	Bottle			
12 AM					
1					
2					
3					
4					
5					
6					
7					
8					
9					
10					
11					
12 PM					
1					
2					
3					
4					
5					
6					
7					
8					
9					
10					
11					
12 AM					

date : ....

	Feeding		Changing	Sleep	Notes
	Breast	Bottle			
12 AM	....	....	....	....	....
1	....	....	....	....	....
2	....	....	....	....	....
3	....	....	....	....	....
4	....	....	....	....	....
5	....	....	....	....	....
6	....	....	....	....	....
7	....	....	....	....	....
8	....	....	....	....	....
9	....	....	....	....	....
10	....	....	....	....	....
11	....	....	....	....	....
12 PM	....	....	....	....	....
1	....	....	....	....	....
2	....	....	....	....	....
3	....	....	....	....	....
4	....	....	....	....	....
5	....	....	....	....	....
6	....	....	....	....	....
7	....	....	....	....	....
8	....	....	....	....	....
9	....	....	....	....	....
10	....	....	....	....	....
11	....	....	....	....	....
12 AM	....	....	....	....	....

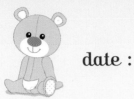

date : ....

	Feeding		Changing	Sleep	Notes
	Breast	Bottle			
12 AM					
1					
2					
3					
4					
5					
6					
7					
8					
9					
10					
11					
12 PM					
1					
2					
3					
4					
5					
6					
7					
8					
9					
10					
11					
12 AM					

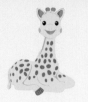

date : ....

	Feeding		Changing	Sleep	Notes
	Breast	Bottle			
12 AM					
1					
2					
3					
4					
5					
6					
7					
8					
9					
10					
11					
12 PM					
1					
2					
3					
4					
5					
6					
7					
8					
9					
10					
11					
12 AM					

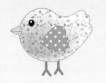

date : ....

	Feeding		Changing	Sleep	Notes
	Breast	Bottle			
12 AM					
1					
2					
3					
4					
5					
6					
7					
8					
9					
10					
11					
12 PM					
1					
2					
3					
4					
5					
6					
7					
8					
9					
10					
11					
12 AM					

date : ....

	Feeding		Changing	Sleep	Notes
	Breast	Bottle			
12 AM					
1					
2					
3					
4					
5					
6					
7					
8					
9					
10					
11					
12 PM					
1					
2					
3					
4					
5					
6					
7					
8					
9					
10					
11					
12 AM					

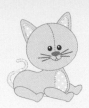

date :

	Feeding		Changing	Sleep	Notes
	Breast	Bottle			
12 AM					
1					
2					
3					
4					
5					
6					
7					
8					
9					
10					
11					
12 PM					
1					
2					
3					
4					
5					
6					
7					
8					
9					
10					
11					
12 AM					

date :

	Feeding		Changing	Sleep	Notes
	Breast	Bottle			
12 AM					
1					
2					
3					
4					
5					
6					
7					
8					
9					
10					
11					
12 PM					
1					
2					
3					
4					
5					
6					
7					
8					
9					
10					
11					
12 AM					

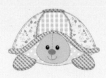

date : ....

	Feeding		Changing	Sleep	Notes
	Breast	Bottle			
12 AM	....	....	....	....	....
1	....	....	....	....	....
2	....	....	....	....	....
3	....	....	....	....	....
4	....	....	....	....	....
5	....	....	....	....	....
6	....	....	....	....	....
7	....	....	....	....	....
8	....	....	....	....	....
9	....	....	....	....	....
10	....	....	....	....	....
11	....	....	....	....	....
12 PM	....	....	....	....	....
1	....	....	....	....	....
2	....	....	....	....	....
3	....	....	....	....	....
4	....	....	....	....	....
5	....	....	....	....	....
6	....	....	....	....	....
7	....	....	....	....	....
8	....	....	....	....	....
9	....	....	....	....	....
10	....	....	....	....	....
11	....	....	....	....	....
12 AM	....	....	....	....	....

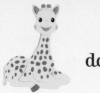

date : ....

	Feeding		Changing	Sleep	Notes
	Breast	Bottle			
12 AM	....	....	....	....	....
1	....	....	....	....	....
2	....	....	....	....	....
3	....	....	....	....	....
4	....	....	....	....	....
5	....	....	....	....	....
6	....	....	....	....	....
7	....	....	....	....	....
8	....	....	....	....	....
9	....	....	....	....	....
10	....	....	....	....	....
11	....	....	....	....	....
12 PM	....	....	....	....	....
1	....	....	....	....	....
2	....	....	....	....	....
3	....	....	....	....	....
4	....	....	....	....	....
5	....	....	....	....	....
6	....	....	....	....	....
7	....	....	....	....	....
8	....	....	....	....	....
9	....	....	....	....	....
10	....	....	....	....	....
11	....	....	....	....	....
12 AM	....	....	....	....	....

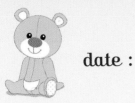

date :

	Feeding		Changing	Sleep	Notes
	Breast	Bottle			
12 AM					
1					
2					
3					
4					
5					
6					
7					
8					
9					
10					
11					
12 PM					
1					
2					
3					
4					
5					
6					
7					
8					
9					
10					
11					
12 AM					

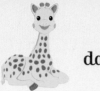

date : ....

	Feeding		Changing	Sleep	Notes
	Breast	Bottle			
12 AM					
1					
2					
3					
4					
5					
6					
7					
8					
9					
10					
11					
12 PM					
1					
2					
3					
4					
5					
6					
7					
8					
9					
10					
11					
12 AM					

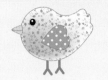

date : ....

	Feeding		Changing	Sleep	Notes
	Breast	Bottle			
12 AM	....	....	....	....	....
1	....	....	....	....	....
2	....	....	....	....	....
3	....	....	....	....	....
4	....	....	....	....	....
5	....	....	....	....	....
6	....	....	....	....	....
7	....	....	....	....	....
8	....	....	....	....	....
9	....	....	....	....	....
10	....	....	....	....	....
11	....	....	....	....	....
12 PM	....	....	....	....	....
1	....	....	....	....	....
2	....	....	....	....	....
3	....	....	....	....	....
4	....	....	....	....	....
5	....	....	....	....	....
6	....	....	....	....	....
7	....	....	....	....	....
8	....	....	....	....	....
9	....	....	....	....	....
10	....	....	....	....	....
11	....	....	....	....	....
12 AM	....	....	....	....	....

date :

	Feeding		Changing	Sleep	Notes
	Breast	Bottle			
12 AM					
1					
2					
3					
4					
5					
6					
7					
8					
9					
10					
11					
12 PM					
1					
2					
3					
4					
5					
6					
7					
8					
9					
10					
11					
12 AM					

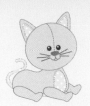

date :

	Feeding		Changing	Sleep	Notes
	Breast	Bottle			
12 AM					
1					
2					
3					
4					
5					
6					
7					
8					
9					
10					
11					
12 PM					
1					
2					
3					
4					
5					
6					
7					
8					
9					
10					
11					
12 AM					

date :

	Feeding		Changing	Sleep	Notes
	Breast	Bottle			
12 AM					
1					
2					
3					
4					
5					
6					
7					
8					
9					
10					
11					
12 PM					
1					
2					
3					
4					
5					
6					
7					
8					
9					
10					
11					
12 AM					

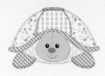

date : ....

	Feeding		Changing	Sleep	Notes
	Breast	Bottle			
12 AM					
1					
2					
3					
4					
5					
6					
7					
8					
9					
10					
11					
12 PM					
1					
2					
3					
4					
5					
6					
7					
8					
9					
10					
11					
12 AM					

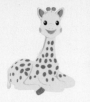

date : ....

	Feeding		Changing	Sleep	Notes
	Breast	Bottle			
12 AM					
1					
2					
3					
4					
5					
6					
7					
8					
9					
10					
11					
12 PM					
1					
2					
3					
4					
5					
6					
7					
8					
9					
10					
11					
12 AM					

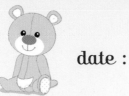

date : ....

	Feeding		Changing	Sleep	Notes
	Breast	Bottle			
12 AM					
1					
2					
3					
4					
5					
6					
7					
8					
9					
10					
11					
12 PM					
1					
2					
3					
4					
5					
6					
7					
8					
9					
10					
11					
12 AM					

date : ....

	Feeding		Changing	Sleep	Notes
	Breast	Bottle			
12 AM					
1					
2					
3					
4					
5					
6					
7					
8					
9					
10					
11					
12 PM					
1					
2					
3					
4					
5					
6					
7					
8					
9					
10					
11					
12 AM					

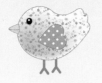

date : ....

	Feeding		Changing	Sleep	Notes
	Breast	Bottle			
12 AM					
1					
2					
3					
4					
5					
6					
7					
8					
9					
10					
11					
12 PM					
1					
2					
3					
4					
5					
6					
7					
8					
9					
10					
11					
12 AM					

date : ....

	Feeding		Changing	Sleep	Notes
	Breast	Bottle			
12 AM					
1					
2					
3					
4					
5					
6					
7					
8					
9					
10					
11					
12 PM					
1					
2					
3					
4					
5					
6					
7					
8					
9					
10					
11					
12 AM					

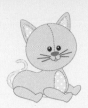

date :

	Feeding		Changing	Sleep	Notes
	Breast	Bottle			
12 AM					
1					
2					
3					
4					
5					
6					
7					
8					
9					
10					
11					
12 PM					
1					
2					
3					
4					
5					
6					
7					
8					
9					
10					
11					
12 AM